The Ultimate

Alkaline Cookbook

Easy and Quick
Alkaline Diet to Reset and
Rebalance your Metabolism

Sam Carter

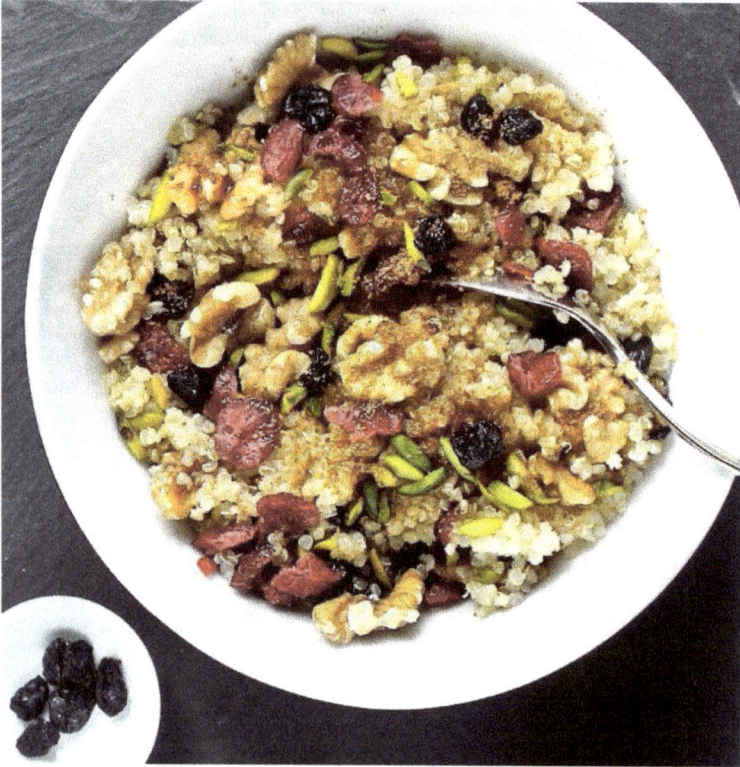

By reading this document, the reader agrees that under no circumstances is the author responsible for any losses, direct or indirect, which are incurred as a result of the use of information contained within this document, including, but not limited to, — errors, omissions, or inaccuracies.

Table of Contents

Three Onion Soup 9

Watermelon, Mint & Tofu Kebabs 12

Blackberry Salsa 14

Smokey Nut Mix 16

Seaweed Spread 18

Spring Soup 20

Herbed Mushrooms 23

Guacamole Hummus 26

Avocado & Tomato Salad 29

Cheesy Zucchini Chips 31

Curry Pepper Hummus 32

Mushroom & Onion Kebabs 35

Open Faced Avocado Sandwich 37

Mediterranean Parsnip Fries 39

Scallion Chickpea Cakes 43

Sweet Chili Carrot Fries 45

Spiced Apple Slices 47

Coconut Butter Dates 48

Warm Avocado Cups 49

Fruit Salsa 51

Chocolate Orange Pineapple Rings 53

Cheesy Bean Chips 57

Banana Strawberry Bites 59

Spinach & Artichoke Stuffed Mushroom 61

Quick Avocado Wraps 64

Strawberry Toast 66

Triple Berry Parfait 67

Sweet & Savory Almonds 68

Plantain Chips 70

Coconut Figgy Toast 71

Tamari Pepitas Snack 73

Green Hummus 74

Spinach Artichoke Dip 76

Spinach Cabbage Soup 78

Fermented Greens 81

Coconut Asparagus Soup 83

Vegetable & Rice Stew 85

Dairy Free Fruity Milk Jar 88

Cleansing Soup 89

Red Citrus Salad 91

Sweet Summer Soup 94

Melon Pie 95

Super Smooth Parsnip Soup 97

Cucumber & Salmon Cups 99

Sweet Potato Toasts 100

Eggplant Cashew Bites 102

Curry Chips 104

Mexican Dip 106

Three Onion Soup

Servings: 2

Total Time: 45 minutes

Ingredients

- 2 tablespoons ghee
- 1 large yellow onion, peeled and thinly sliced
- 1 large leek, sliced
- ¼ cup green onions, sliced
- 3 small potatoes, quartered
- 2 garlic cloves, minced
- 3 cups vegetable broth
- 1 teaspoon Himalayan salt
- 1 teaspoon black pepper, crushed

Directions

1.   In a large stockpot over medium heat, add ghee, yellow onions, leeks and green onions. Cook 10-15 minutes, lightly caramelizing the onions.

2.   Add potatoes, garlic and broth. Bring to a boil and then reduce heat to low and simmer 25 minutes or until potatoes are tender.

3.   Season with salt and pepper before serving.

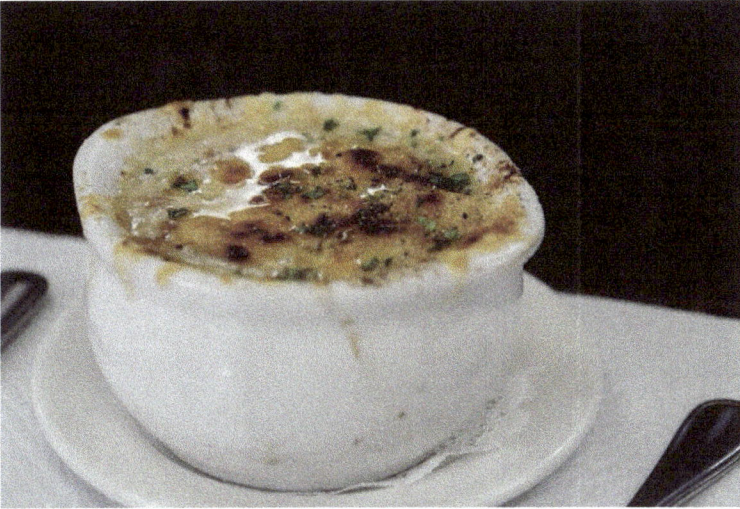

Watermelon, Mint & Tofu Kebabs

Servings: 2

Total Time: 10 minutes

Ingredients

- 8 watermelon cubes
- 8 tofu cubes
- 8 mint leaves
- 1 tablespoon olive oil
- 1 teaspoon Himalayan salt
- 1 teaspoon black pepper, crushed
- 4 bamboo skewers, cut in half

Directions

1. On each skewer, place a watermelon cube, tofu cube and a mint leaf.

2. Drizzle each skewer with olive oil and sprinkle with salt and pepper

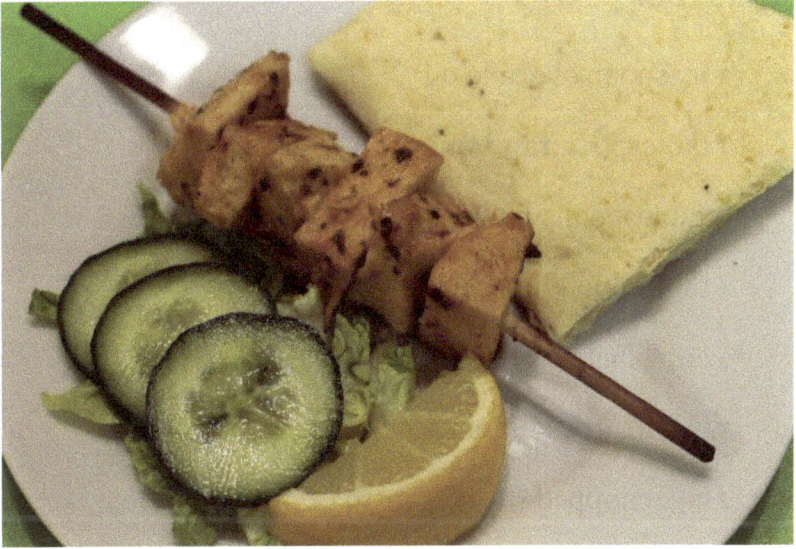

Blackberry Salsa

Servings: 2

Total Time: 15 minutes

Ingredients

- 1 teaspoon avocado oil

- 1 tablespoon raw honey

- 3 tablespoons lime juice

- 1 tablespoon lime zest

- 1 cup blackberries

- 1/3 cup green onions, chopped

- 1 cup chopped fresh cilantro

- 1 jalapeno, seeded and diced

- ¼ cup pumpkin seeds, toasted

- ¼ teaspoon Himalayan salt

Directions

1.   Whisk together the avocado oil, honey, lime juice and lime zest in a small bowl.

2.   In a large bowl, muddle the blackberries gently with the end of a spoon. Add in green onions, cilantro, jalapeno and pumpkin seeds.

3.   Pour oil and honey mixture over the blackberries. Season with salt and toss to combine.

4.   Chill 10 minutes before serving with cut up vegetables.

Smokey Nut Mix

Servings: 2

Total Time: 10 minutes

Ingredients

- 1 teaspoon coconut oil

- 2 tablespoons honey

- 1 tablespoon coconut aminos

- ½ cup pecans

- ½ cup almonds

- ½ teaspoon cinnamon

- ¼ teaspoon cayenne pepper

- ⅛ teaspoon smoked paprika

Directions

1. In a small bowl, combine all the ingredients and make sure the nuts are well coated.

2. Preheat oven to 300°F/150°C and line a baking tray with parchment paper.

3.   Spread nuts on the baking tray and ensure they are in a single layer.

4.   Place baking tray in the oven and cook for 5 minutes, stirring frequently to ensure they do not burn.

5.   Remove and let cool in a small bowl.

Seaweed Spread

Servings: 2

Total Time: 10 minutes

Ingredients

- 1 cup cashews, soaked overnight and drained
- 1 teaspoon dried dulse seaweed
- 1 teaspoon dried wakame
- 1 garlic clove, minced
- 1 teaspoon black pepper, crushed
- ½ lemon, juiced
- ½ teaspoon dill, chopped
- ½ teaspoon Himalayan salt
- 1 tablespoon apple cider vinegar
- ¼ cucumber, chopped
- 4 teaspoons red onion, minced
- ½ cup celery, minced

Directions

1.   Blend the first 9 ingredients together in a food processor until smooth but still with some texture.

2.   Transfer to medium sized bowl and fold in the cucumber, red onion and celery.

3.   Serve with cut up vegetables or gluten-free crackers.

Spring Soup

Servings: 2

Total Time: 35 minutes

Ingredients

- 1 tablespoon olive oil

- 2 shallots, sliced

- 1 cup asparagus, trimmed and cut into 1-inch pieces

- ½ cup artichoke hearts

- 1 garlic clove, minced

- 1 ½ cups vegetable broth

- ¼ cup water

- 1 teaspoon apple cider vinegar

- ½ teaspoon oregano

- ¼ teaspoon turmeric

- ¼ teaspoon cayenne pepper

- ½ teaspoon Himalayan salt

- ½ teaspoon black pepper, crushed

- ½ lemon, juiced

- 1 tablespoon chives

Directions

1.   In a medium saucepan over medium heat, add oil, shallots, asparagus, artichoke and garlic. Cook 8 minutes and then add the broth, water, vinegar, oregano, turmeric, cayenne, salt and pepper.

2.   Bring to a boil and then reduce heat to low and simmer 15 minutes.

3.   Let cool slightly and transfer to a food processor or blender. Blend until mixture is smooth.

4.   Place back in the saucepan over medium-low heat and bring to a simmer before stirring in lemon juice.

5.   Garnish with chives before serving.

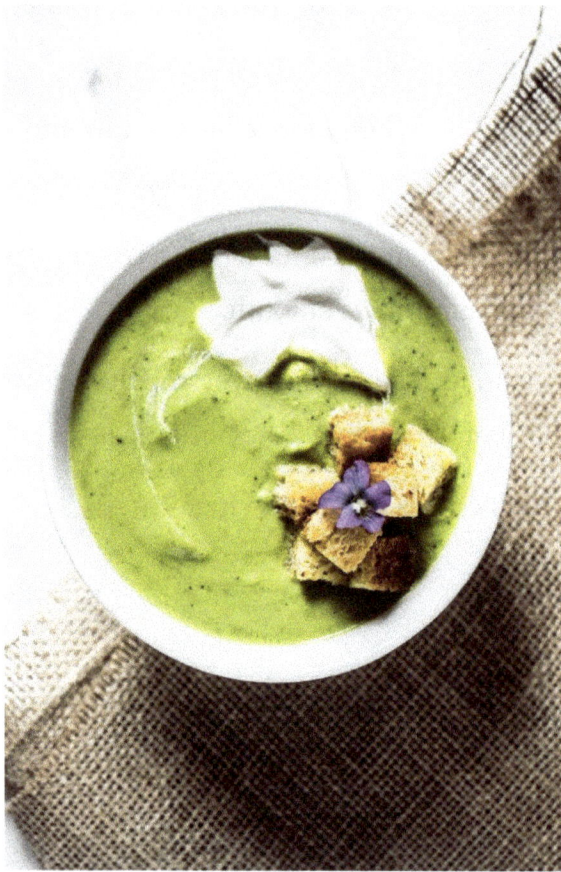

Herbed Mushrooms

Servings: 2 (5 mushrooms each)

Total Time: 20 minutes

Ingredients

- 1 cup cashews, soaked 3 hours then drained and rinsed
- 1 garlic clove, chopped
- 1 tablespoon lemon juice
- ½ teaspoon Himalayan salt
- ½ cup silken tofu
- 1 tablespoon nutritional yeast
- ¼ teaspoon cayenne pepper
- ¼ cup fresh dill, chopped
- ¼ cup fresh parsley, chopped
- ¼ teaspoon black pepper, crushed
- 10 mushrooms, stems removed
- 5 cherry tomatoes, halved

Directions

1.   Preheat oven to 350°F/180°C. Line a baking tray with parchment paper.

2.   Place cashews, garlic, lemon juice, salt and tofu in a food processor and blend until well combined and smooth.

3.   Add nutritional yeast, cayenne, dill, parsley and pepper to the food processor and blend until incorporated.

4.   Stuff each mushroom with the cashew mixture and top with half a tomato.

5.   Bake in the oven for 15 minutes or until mushrooms are soft.

6.   Serve immediately.

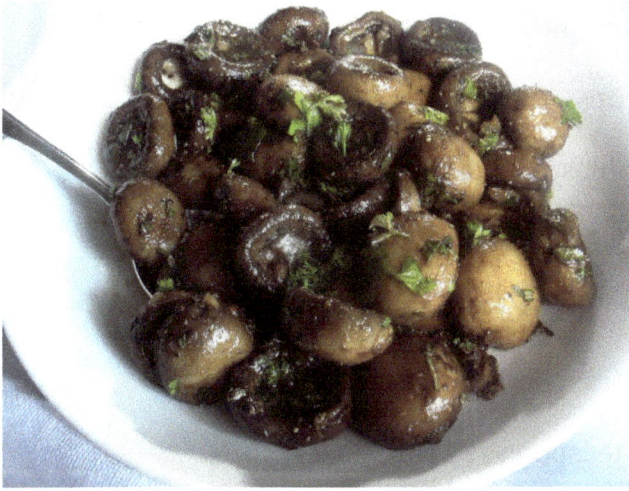

Guacamole Hummus

Servings: 2

Total Time: 5 minutes

Ingredients

- 2 avocados
- 2 cups of chickpeas, cooked
- 1 tablespoon tahini
- 1 garlic clove, minced
- 3 tablespoons lemon juice
- ½ teaspoon cumin
- ½ teaspoon red chili flakes
- 1 tablespoon avocado oil
- ½ teaspoon Himalayan salt
- ¼ teaspoon black pepper, crushed
- 2 tablespoons cilantro, chopped
- 1 cucumber, sliced
- 1 carrot, cut into sticks

Directions

1. Combine all ingredients, except cucumber and carrots, in a food processor until smooth.

2. Serve with cucumbers and carrots

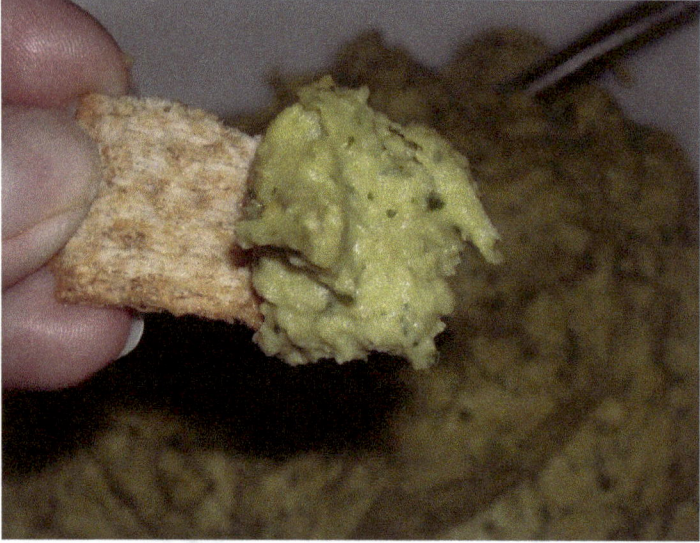

Avocado & Tomato Salad

Servings: 2

Total Time: 5 minutes

Ingredients

- 2 avocados, diced
- 4 Roma tomatoes, quartered
- ¼ cup red onion, thinly sliced
- 2 tablespoons cilantro
- ½ teaspoon Himalayan salt
- ½ teaspoon black pepper, crushed

Directions

1.   Combine all ingredients in a medium-sized bowl and toss well.

2.   Serve immediately either on its own or with some crackers.

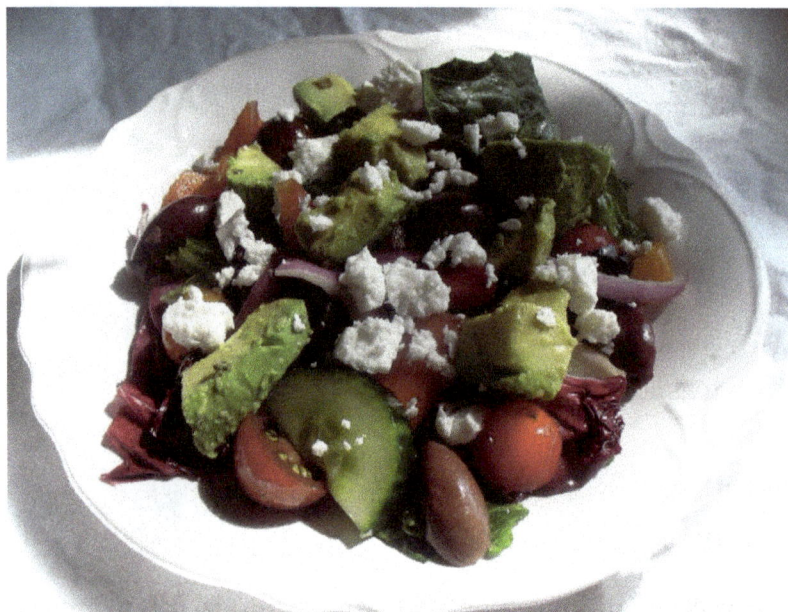

Cheesy Zucchini Chips

Servings: 2

Total Time: 5 minutes plus 2 hours bake time

Ingredients

- 1 large zucchini, sliced thinly
- 2 tablespoons olive oil
- 1 teaspoon Himalayan salt
- 2 teaspoons onion powder
- 1 teaspoon garlic powder
- 2 tablespoons nutritional yeast

Directions

1. Preheat oven to 200°F/95°C. Line a baking tray with a parchment paper.

2. Toss all ingredients in a large bowl so that the zucchini is evenly coated.

3. Place on baking tray and bake for 2 hours or until crispy.

Curry Pepper Hummus

Servings: 2

Total Time: 5 minutes plus 2 hours bake time

Ingredients

- 1 red bell pepper

- 2 tablespoons olive oil

- ½ cup chickpeas

- 1 tablespoon tahini

- 1 garlic clove

- ½ lemon, juiced

- ½ teaspoon Himalayan salt

- ½ teaspoon curry powder

- ¼ teaspoon turmeric

- ¼ teaspoon chili flakes

- 1 teaspoon cilantro

- 1 cucumber, sliced

- 1 carrot, cut into sticks

Directions

1.   Place all ingredients except the cilantro, cucumber and carrot into a food processor and blend until smooth.

2.   Garnish with cilantro and serve with cucumber and carrot.

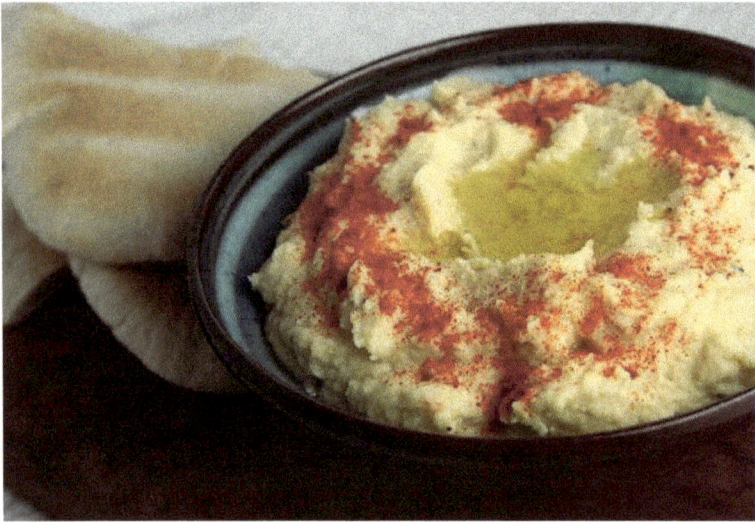

Mushroom & Onion Kebabs

Servings: 2

Total Time: 35 minutes

Ingredients

- 2 tablespoons olive oil
- 1 garlic clove, minced
- 1-inch piece ginger, grated
- ½ tablespoon tamari
- ½ tablespoon coconut aminos
- 1 teaspoon lime juice
- 1 teaspoon lime zest
- ½ tablespoon red chili flakes
- 15 cremini mushrooms, stems removed and sliced
- ½ red onion, quartered
- ½ teaspoon Himalayan salt
- 4 bamboo skewers, soaked 15 minutes
- 1 tablespoon cilantro, chopped

Directions

1.   Place olive oil, garlic, ginger, tamari, coconut aminos, lime juice, lime zest and red chili flakes in a medium bowl. Whisk together well and add mushrooms, onion and salt.

2.   Let mushrooms and onions sit for 15 minutes and then place on the skewers in alternating pattern.

3.   Heat a grill pan over medium-high heat and grill mushroom skewers for 5 minutes on each side.

4.   Garnish with cilantro and serve immediately.

Open Faced Avocado Sandwich

Servings: 2

Total Time: 5 minutes

Ingredients

- 2 slices sprouted bread, toasted

- 2 tablespoons hummus, divided

- 1 ripe avocado, sliced and divided

- 4 tomato slices

- 4 cucumber slices

- 1 tablespoon sunflower seeds

- 1 teaspoon nutritional yeast

- ½ teaspoon Himalayan salt

- ½ teaspoon black pepper, crushed

Directions

1. Top each slice of toast with hummus, avocado, 2 tomato slices, 2 cucumber slices, sunflower seeds, nutritional yeast, salt and pepper.

2. Serve immediately.

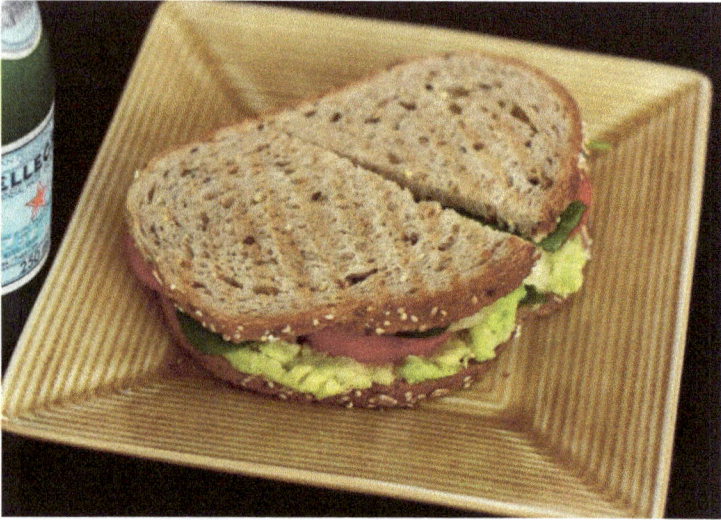

Mediterranean Parsnip Fries

Servings: 2

Total Time: 25 minutes

Ingredients

- 5 parsnips, cut into strips or wedges
- 2 tablespoons olive oil
- 2 garlic cloves, minced
- 1 teaspoon dried oregano
- 1 teaspoon dried thyme
- 1 teaspoon dried basil
- 1 teaspoon onion powder

Directions

1. Preheat oven to 400°F/205°C. Line a baking tray with parchment paper.

2. Add all the ingredients to a medium-sized bowl and toss well to coat.

3. Lay parsnips on a baking tray in an even layer.

4. Bake in the oven for 20 minutes or until crispy.

Spicy Sweet Potato Bites

Servings: 2

Total Time: 30 minutes

Ingredients

- 1 small and narrow sweet potato, sliced into thin slices
- 1 teaspoon olive oil
- ½ teaspoon cayenne pepper
- ¼ teaspoon smoked paprika
- ¼ teaspoon garlic powder
- ¼ teaspoon Himalayan salt
- 1 avocado, mashed
- ¼ cup tomato, diced
- 1 garlic clove, minced
- 1 shallot, diced
- ½ lime, juiced
- 1 tablespoon cilantro, chopped

Directions

1.	Preheat oven to 400°F/205°C. Line a baking tray with parchment paper.

2.	Add the sweet potato, olive oil, cayenne, paprika, garlic powder and salt to a medium-sized bowl and toss well to coat.

3.	Lay sweet potatoes on baking tray in an even layer. Bake in the oven for 20 minutes or until crispy.

4.	While sweet potatoes are in the oven, combine the avocado, tomato, garlic, shallot, lime and cilantro in a medium-sized bowl until well combined.

5.	Remove sweet potatoes from the oven and let cool for 5 minutes.

6.	Top with avocado mixture and serve.

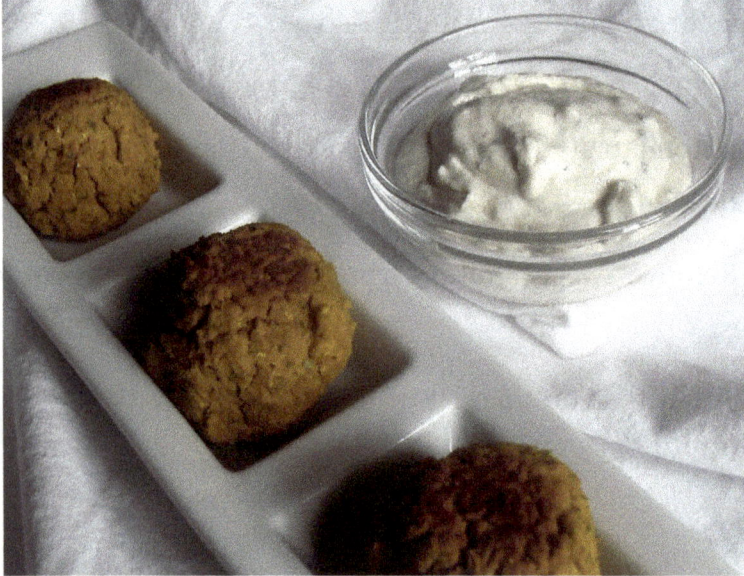

Scallion Chickpea Cakes

Servings: 2

Total Time: 20 minutes

Ingredients

- ¾ cup chickpea flour
- ½ cup water
- ¼ teaspoon garlic powder
- ½ teaspoon Himalayan salt
- ½ teaspoon black pepper, crushed
- 2 shallots, diced
- ½ cup green onion, sliced
- 2 tablespoons, cilantro
- 1 tablespoon coconut oil
- 2 tablespoons tamari
- 1 tablespoon coconut aminos
- 1 teaspoon chives, chopped

Directions

1.   Combine all the ingredients, except the coconut oil, tamari, coconut aminos and chives in a medium-sized mixing bowl and stir until combined to form the batter.

2.   Heat coconut oil in a medium skillet over medium-high heat. Add two tablespoons of batter to the skillet in a circular shape. Let cook 4-5 minutes or until browned on the bottom and flip.

3.   Cook another 4 minutes and then remove.

4.   Combine the tamari and coconut aminos in a small dish.

5.   Garnish the cakes with the chives and serve with tamari sauce.

Sweet Chili Carrot Fries

Servings: 2

Total Time: 30 minutes

Ingredients

- 8 large carrots, cut into wedges
- 1 tablespoon avocado oil
- 1 teaspoon garlic powder
- ½ teaspoon Himalayan salt
- ½ teaspoon cayenne pepper
- ¼ teaspoon coconut sugar

Chili Sauce

- 2 tablespoons coconut aminos
- 1 tablespoon honey
- 1 teaspoon red chili flakes

Directions

1. Preheat oven to 400°F/205°C. Line a baking tray with parchment paper.

2.   Place carrots, oil, garlic, salt, cayenne and coconut sugar in a large mixing bowl and toss well to coat.

3.   Lay carrots on a baking tray in an even layer and bake in the oven for 25 minutes or until crispy.

4.   While carrots bake, mix together the Chili Sauce ingredients in a small bowl.

5.   Remove carrots and serve with Chili Sauce.

Spiced Apple Slices

Servings: 2

Total Time: 5 minutes

Ingredients

- 1 red apple, core removed and sliced into circular slices
- ½ teaspoon lemon juice
- 3 tablespoons cashew butter
- 1 tablespoon raisins
- 1 tablespoon sunflower seeds
- ½ teaspoon cinnamon powder

Directions

1. Place apple slices on a plate and drizzle with the lemon juice (to prevent browning).

2. Spread cashew butter on each of the apple slices and then top with raisins, sunflower seeds and cinnamon powder.

3. Serve immediately.

Coconut Butter Dates

Servings: 2

Total Time: 5 minutes

Ingredients

- 10 dates, pitted
- 2 tablespoons coconut butter

Directions

1. Stuff each date with some of the coconut butter.

2. Chill 10 minutes before serving.

Warm Avocado Cups

Servings: 2

Total Time: 8 minutes

Ingredients

- 1 ripe avocado, pitted
- 1 teaspoon coconut oil
- ¼ teaspoon cayenne pepper
- 2 tablespoons honey
- 1 tablespoon coconut aminos
- ¼ cup pepitas, toasted
- 1 tablespoon cilantro, chopped

Directions

1. Brush coconut oil on each open side of the avocado and then sprinkle with cayenne.

2. Heat grill pan over medium-high heat and add avocado, keep the cut side facing down. Cook 5 minutes or until lightly grilled.

3. Remove avocados from pan, drizzle with honey and coconut aminos and then top with pepitas and cilantro.

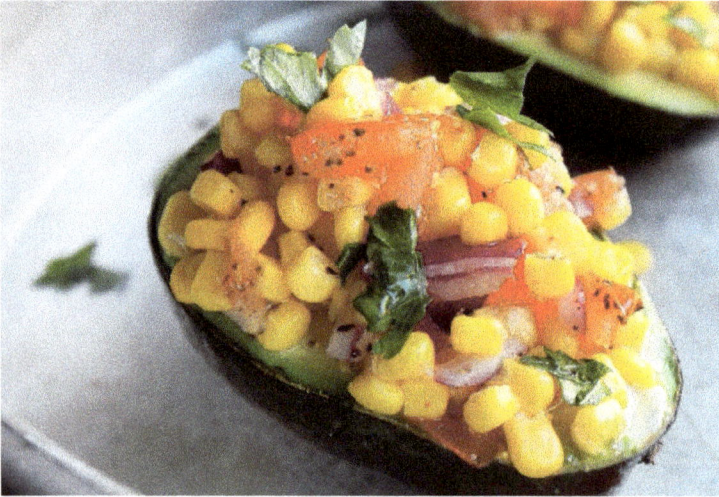

Fruit Salsa

Servings: 2

Total Time: 25 minutes

Ingredients

- ½ pineapple, finely chopped
- ½ cucumber, finely chopped
- ½ mango, finely chopped
- ½ green bell pepper, finely chopped
- ¼ cup green onion, sliced
- 2 limes, zested and juiced
- 1/3 cup cilantro, roughly chopped
- 1 teaspoon cayenne pepper
- ½ teaspoon Himalayan salt
- ½ teaspoon coconut aminos
- 1 cup sprouted tortilla chips or crackers

Directions

1.   Combine all ingredients, except the chips in a medium mixing bowl.

2.   Let sit in the fridge for 20 minutes before serving with tortilla chips.

Chocolate Orange Pineapple Rings

Servings: 2

Total Time: 10 minutes plus 30 minutes chill time

Ingredients

- ¼ cup coconut oil
- 2 tablespoons cacao powder
- 1 tablespoon maple syrup
- 10 dried pineapple rings
- 1 tablespoon unsweetened, shredded coconut
- 1 teaspoon almonds, slivered
- 1 teaspoon cacao nibs
- 1 teaspoon orange zest
- ¼ teaspoon Himalayan salt

Directions

1. In a small bowl, combine coconut oil, cacao and maple syrup to create the chocolate mixture.

2. Line a baking tray with parchment paper.

3.   Dip half of a pineapple ring in chocolate mixture. Lay on baking tray and sprinkle with some of the coconut, almonds, cacao nibs, orange zest and salt (sprinkle on the chocolate side).

4.   Repeat with remaining pineapple rings and toppings.

5.   Chill 30 minutes in the fridge before serving.

Raspberry Mint Yogurt Pops

Servings: 2

Total Time: 5 minutes plus 2 hours chill time

Ingredients

- 1 teaspoon honey

- 2 cups unsweetened yogurt

- ¼ cup mint, finely chopped

- ½ cup raspberries

Directions

1. In a small bowl, combine the honey, yogurt and mint.

2. Place a few raspberries in the bottom of 4 popsicle molds. Add in some of the yogurt mixture and then add a few more raspberries. Top each mold with remaining yogurt mixture.

3. Place in the freezer for at least 2 hours.

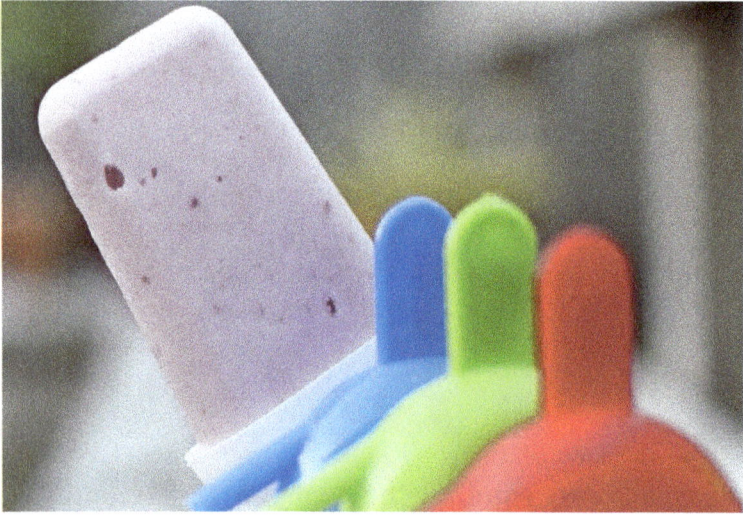

Cheesy Bean Chips

Servings: 2

Total Time: 35 minutes

Ingredients

- 3 cups green beans
- ¼ cup avocado oil
- 2 teaspoon Himalayan salt
- ¼ cup nutritional yeast
- 1 teaspoon garlic powder
- 1 teaspoon onion powder
- 1 teaspoon paprika
- ½ teaspoon cayenne pepper

Directions

1. Preheat oven to 400°F/205°C. Line a baking tray with parchment paper.

2. Toss all ingredients in a medium-sized bowl to properly coat the green beans.

3.   Place green beans on the baking tray and bake in the oven 30 minutes or until crispy.

Banana Strawberry Bites

Servings: 2

Total Time: 10 minutes plus 1 hour freeze time

Ingredients

- 2 large bananas, sliced into ½ inch pieces
- 1/3 cup almond butter
- 3 strawberries, sliced
- 3 tablespoons coconut oil, melted
- 1 tablespoon raw cacao powder
- 1 teaspoon maple syrup
- ¼ teaspoon Himalayan salt

Directions

1. Take a banana slice and spread each slice with some almond butter. Top with a strawberry slice and then put a banana slice on top to make a sandwich.

2. In a small bowl, combine the oil, cacao, maple syrup and salt to form the chocolate mixture.

3. Dip each banana sandwich in the chocolate mixture and place on a parchment paper lined baking tray.

4.   Freeze at least 1 hour in the freezer before serving.

Spinach & Artichoke Stuffed Mushroom

Servings: 2

Total Time: 20 minutes

Ingredients

- 6 white button mushrooms, stems removed and chopped (keep the remaining head of the mushroom)
- 1 cup spinach, steamed and chopped
- ¼ cup canned artichoke, drained and chopped
- ¼ cup nutritional yeast
- 1 tablespoon olive oil
- ¼ teaspoon garlic powder
- ¼ teaspoon onion
- ⅛ teaspoon pepper
- ¼ teaspoon Himalayan salt

Directions

1. Add the mushroom stems, spinach, artichoke, nutritional yeast, olive oil, garlic, onion, pepper and salt to a food processor. Pulse a few times until combined but not entirely smooth.

2.   Preheat oven to 350°F/180°C and line a baking tray with parchment paper.

3.   Stuff each mushroom head with the spinach and artichoke mixture and place on the parchment paper.

4.   Bake for 15 minutes.

5.   Remove and serve hot.

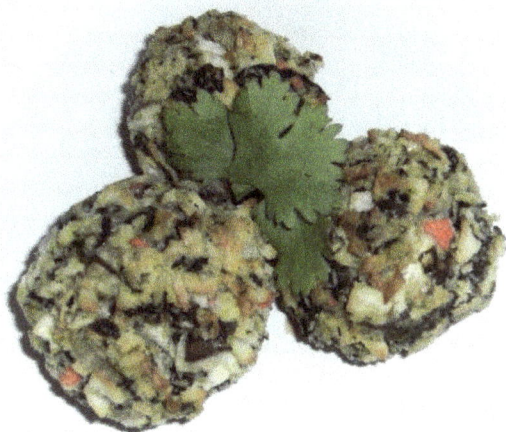

Quick Avocado Wraps

Servings: 2

Total Time: 5 minutes

Ingredients

- 4 Romaine lettuce leaves
- 1 avocado, sliced
- 1 ½ cups sprouts
- ½ cup hummus
- 1 cucumber, sliced
- 1 tablespoon sunflower seeds
- ¼ teaspoon Himalayan salt
- ¼ teaspoon black pepper, crushed

Directions

1. Stuff each lettuce leaf with the avocado, sprouts, hummus, cucumber, sunflower seeds, salt and pepper.

2. Roll up and enjoy.

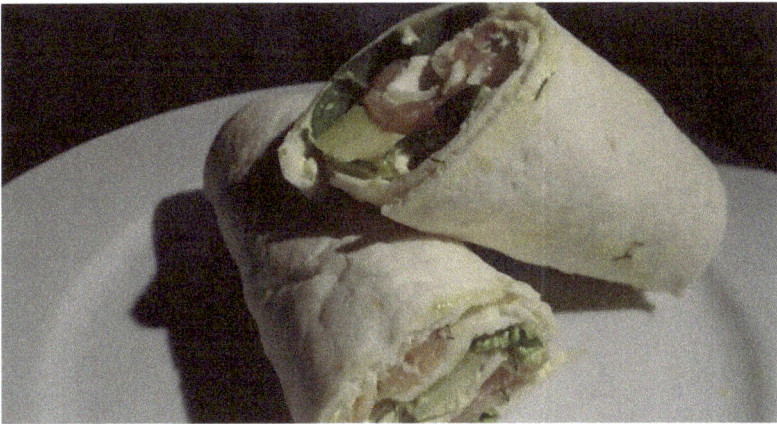

Strawberry Toast

Servings: 2

Total Time: 5 minutes

Ingredients

- 2 slices sprouted bread, toasted
- 3 tablespoons almond butter
- 2 tablespoons unsweetened yogurt
- 4 strawberries, hulled and sliced
- ½ teaspoon cinnamon
- 1 tablespoon chia seeds
- 1 tablespoon sunflower seeds

Directions

1. Spread almond butter on each of the slices of toast.

2. Top with yogurt, sliced strawberries, cinnamon, chia seeds and sunflower seeds.

3. Serve immediately.

Triple Berry Parfait

Servings: 2

Total Time: 5 minutes

Ingredients

- ½ cup strawberries, hulled, sliced and divided
- ½ cup raspberries, divided
- ½ cup blueberries, divided
- 1 tablespoon chia seeds
- 1 ½ cups unsweetened yogurt
- 2 tablespoons mint, chopped
- 3 tablespoons almonds, slivered

Directions

1. Layer strawberries in the bottom of two tall glasses. Top with half the chia seeds and then a quarter of the yogurt.

2. Top with half raspberries and a half the almonds.

3. Top with half blueberries and half mint.

4. Repeat with remaining glass and ingredients.

Sweet & Savory Almonds

Servings: 2

Total Time: 30 minutes

Ingredients

- 1 cup raw almonds

- 2 tablespoons raw honey

- 1 tablespoon coconut aminos

- 1 tablespoon tamari

- ½ tablespoon garlic powder

- ½ tablespoon onion powder

- ½ teaspoon celery salt

Directions

1. Preheat oven to 350°F/180°C. Line baking tray with parchment paper.

2. Toss all the ingredients in a medium bowl until well coated.

3. Place almonds on baking tray in an even layer.

4.   Bake in the oven for 25 minutes, stirring every 5 minutes so almonds don't burn.

Plantain Chips

Servings: 2

Total Time: 25 minutes

Ingredients

- 2 large green plantains, sliced
- 1 tablespoon coconut oil
- ½ tablespoon Himalayan salt
- ¼ teaspoon onion powder

Directions

1. Preheat oven to 350°F/180°C. Line baking tray with parchment paper.

2. Toss all the ingredients in a medium-sized bowl until well coated.

3. Add plantain slices to baking tray and bake in the oven for 20 minutes, flipping once after 10 minutes until they are cooked properly to create the "plantain chips."

4. Remove and let cool before serving.

Coconut Figgy Toast

Servings: 2

Total Time: 5 minutes

Ingredients

- 2 sliced sprouted bread, toasted

- 2 tablespoons coconut butter

- 3 fresh figs, sliced

- 1 tablespoon unsweetened, shredded coconut

- 1 teaspoon chia seeds

Directions

1. Spread coconut butter on top of cooled toast slices. Place figs on top of each slice.

2. Sprinkle with shredded coconut and chia seeds.

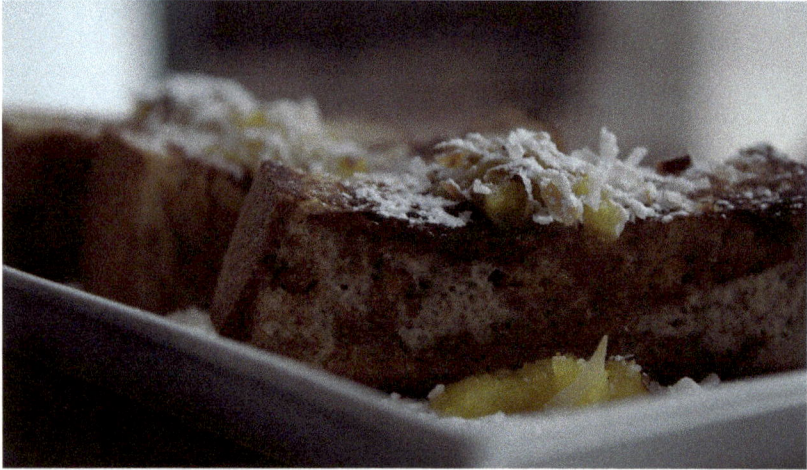

Tamari Pepitas Snack

Servings: 2

Total Time: 25 minutes

Ingredients

- ½ cup pepitas
- 2 tablespoons tamari
- ½ teaspoon coconut aminos
- 1 teaspoon garlic powder
- ½ teaspoon cayenne pepper

Directions

1. Preheat oven to 350°F/180°C. Line baking tray with parchment paper.

2. Toss all the ingredients in a medium-sized bowl until well coated.

3. Add pepitas to baking tray and bake in the oven for 20 minutes, stirring every 5 minutes

4. Remove and let cool before serving. Great to keep in a ziplock bag and snack on throughout the day.

Green Hummus

Servings: 2

Total Time: 5 minutes

Ingredients

- 1 garlic clove

- 2 tablespoons green onion, sliced

- 1 cup chickpeas, drained and rinsed

- 2 tablespoons lemon juice

- ½ cup parsley, chopped

- 1 cup spinach, chopped

- 1 tablespoon cup tahini

- 2 tablespoons olive oil

- 2 tablespoons water

- 1 teaspoon cumin

- 1 teaspoon cayenne pepper

- ½ teaspoon Himalayan salt

- ¼ teaspoon black pepper

- 2 carrot, cut into sticks

- 2 celery stalks, trimmed and cut in half

Directions

1.   In a food processor or blender, combine all ingredients except the carrots and celery to create the hummus. Add more water if mixture is too thick.

2.   Transfer to a small bowl and serve with carrots and celery.

Spinach Artichoke Dip

Servings: 2

Total Time: 5 minutes

Ingredients

- 1 14 ounce can of artichoke hearts
- 2 cups spinach, chopped
- 1 15 ounce can of chickpeas
- 2 tablespoons parsley, chopped
- 4 tablespoons olive oil
- 1 lemon, juiced
- 2 garlic cloves, minced
- 4 tablespoons nutritional yeast
- 1 teaspoon chili powder
- 1 teaspoon paprika
- 1 teaspoon Himalayan salt
- 1 teaspoon black pepper, crushed
- 2 carrot, cut into sticks
- 2 celery stalks, trimmed and cut in half

Directions

1.   Combine all ingredients except the carrots and celery in a food processor or blender and combine until well combined (but still able to see pieces of artichoke and spinach) to create the dip.

2.   Serve with carrots and celery.

Spinach Cabbage Soup

Servings: 2

Total Time: 30 minutes

Ingredients

- 1 tablespoon olive oil
- ¼ cup red onion, diced
- 1 garlic clove, minced
- 1 celery stalk, diced
- 1 medium carrot, diced
- ½ cup mushrooms
- ½ head of broccoli, cut into florets
- ½ cup red bell pepper, diced
- 1 teaspoon fresh ginger, peeled and minced
- ½ turmeric
- ⅛ teaspoon cayenne pepper
- 1 teaspoon Himalayan salt
- 1 teaspoon black pepper, crushed
- 3 ½ cups vegetable broth
- 2 cups spinach, roughly chopped

- ½ cup purple cabbage, thinly shredded

- ¼ cup parsley, chopped

Directions

1. In a large pot, heat olive oil over medium heat. Add onion, garlic, celery and carrot. Cook 5 minutes and then add mushrooms, broccoli, pepper and ginger. Cook an additional 10 minutes.

2. Sprinkle vegetables with turmeric, cayenne, salt and pepper. Cook for 1 minute and add vegetable broth.

3. Bring to a boil then reduce heat and simmer 10 minutes.

4. Stir in spinach, cabbage and parsley, cook another minute and then serve immediately.

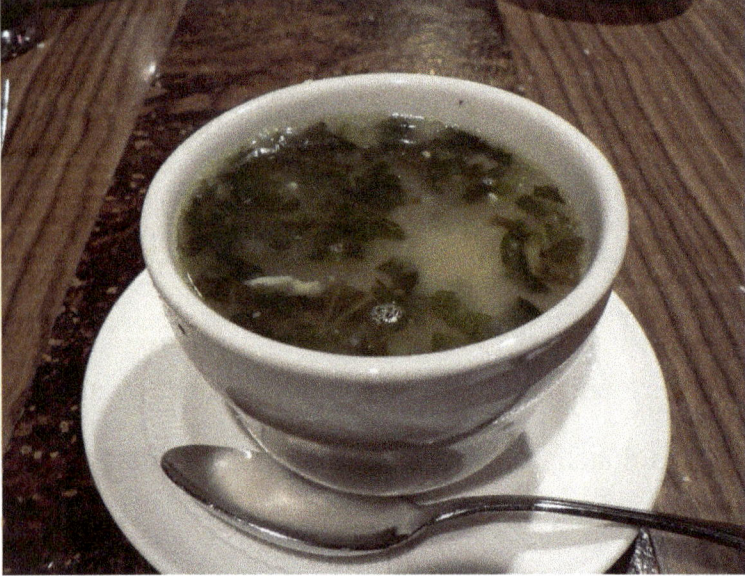

Fermented Greens

Servings: 2

Total Time: 30 minutes (plus 3 days of fermenting)

Ingredients

- 1 cup cabbage, thinly sliced
- 1 cup kale, stems removed and thinly sliced
- 1 cup cucumber, diced
- ½ cup carrot, shredded
- 2 tablespoons green onions, thinly sliced
- 2 tablespoons Himalayan salt
- 1 garlic clove, grated
- 1 tablespoon ginger, grated
- 1 teaspoon cayenne pepper
- 1 tablespoon red chili flakes
- 1 tablespoon smoked paprika
- 2 cups water

Directions

1.   In a large bowl combine the cabbage, kale, cucumber, carrot and green onion. Add salt and massage for 5 minutes, making sure to squeeze vegetables during the 5 minutes.

2.   In a sterilized jar with a lid, add the vegetable mix with the remaining ingredients.

3.   Place jar on a counter in a cool, shaded area for at least 3 days.

4.   Put in fridge after 3 days and chill for a few hours before servings.

Coconut Asparagus Soup

Servings: 2

Total Time: 20 minutes

Ingredients

- 1 tablespoon coconut oil

- 1 shallot, sliced

- 1 garlic clove, minced

- 1 tablespoon green curry paste

- 1 15 ounce can coconut milk

- 1 cup water

- 2 cups asparagus, trimmed and chopped into 1 inch pieces

- 1 cup baby spinach, chopped

- 1 teaspoon Himalayan salt

- 1 teaspoon black pepper, crushed

- 1 tablespoon lime juice

- 1 tablespoon green onions, sliced

- 1 tablespoon cilantro, chopped

Directions

1.   In a large saucepan over medium heat add coconut oil, shallot and garlic. Cook 3 minutes and then add the curry paste. Cook an additional 1 minute.

2.   Pour in the coconut milk, water and asparagus. Bring to a boil and then reduce heat to low and simmer for 15 minutes.

3.   Stir in spinach, salt and pepper. Using an immersion blender, blend mixture until smooth. Stir in lime juice.

4.   Garnish with green onion and cilantro.

Vegetable & Rice Stew

Serving Size: 2

Total Time: 20 minutes

Ingredients

- 1 teaspoon olive oil
- 1 green onion, thinly sliced
- 1 garlic clove, minced
- 1 carrot, sliced into coins
- 1 celery stalk, sliced
- 1 cup white mushrooms, sliced
- ½ cup leeks, sliced
- ¼ cup brown rice
- 2 cups baby kale
- 3 cups vegetable broth
- 1 teaspoon Himalayan salt
- 1 teaspoon black pepper, crushed
- 1 teaspoon dried oregano
- ¼ teaspoon red chili flakes
- ¼ cup fresh parsley, chopped

Directions

1.   Heat olive oil in a large saucepan over medium heat. Add onion, garlic, carrot, celery, mushrooms and leeks. Cook 10 minutes.

2.   Stir in rice and kale and cook 1 minute before adding vegetable broth. Let it come to a boil then reduce heat to low and simmer 15 minutes.

3.   Season with salt, pepper, oregano and chili flakes.

4.   Before serving, stir in parsley.

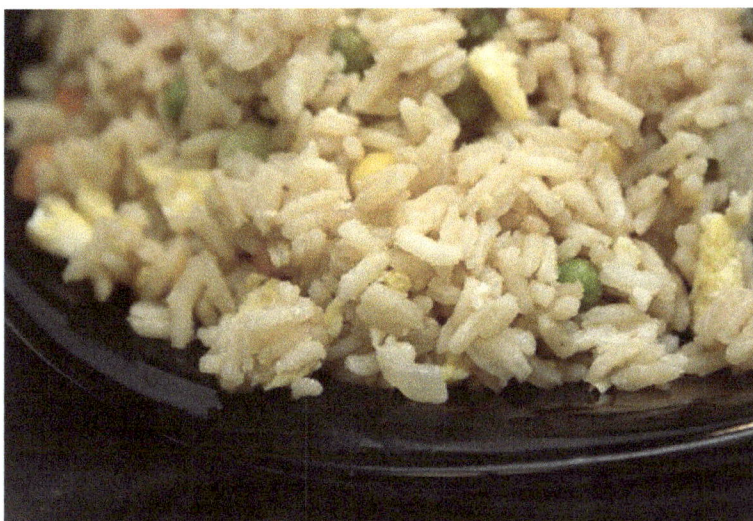

Dairy Free Fruity Milk Jar

Serving Size: 1

Total Time: 15 minutes

Ingredients

- ½ cup raspberries

- 1 teaspoon mint, chopped

- 1 teaspoon raw honey

- ¼ cup chia seeds

- 1 cup unsweetened almond milk

Directions

1.   In a medium sized jar, add raspberries, mint and honey. Mash with the handle of a wooden spoon.

2.   Add chia seeds and almond milk and stir to combine.

3.   Let sit for 10 minutes before serving.

Cleansing Soup

Serving Size: 2

Total Time: 25 minutes

Ingredients

- 1 tablespoon avocado oil
- 1 shallot, sliced
- 2 garlic cloves, sliced
- 1 inch ginger, sliced
- ½ teaspoon ground cumin
- ¼ teaspoon ground turmeric
- 1 ½ cups zucchini, zucchini
- 1 cup broccoli, florets trimmed
- 1 cup spinach
- ½ cup green bell pepper, seeds removed and chopped
- 3 cups water
- 1 teaspoon Himalayan salt
- 1 lemon, zested and juiced
- 2 tablespoons parsley

Directions

1.   Heat oil over medium heat in a large saucepan. Add shallot, garlic, ginger, cumin, turmeric and cook for 5 minutes. Add in zucchini, broccoli, spinach and bell pepper.

2.   Cook another 8 minutes before stirring in the water, salt and lemon juice. Let cook another 5 minutes or until the vegetables are tender.

3.   Place vegetable mixture in a blender or food processor and add the lemon zest and parsley. Blend until smooth and serve warm.

Red Citrus Salad

Serving Size: 2

Total Time: 10 minutes

Ingredients

- 1 tablespoon cup coconut aminos
- ¼ cup apple cider vinegar
- 3 tablespoons orange zest
- 2 tablespoons orange juice
- 1 tablespoon maple syrup
- 1 tablespoon olive oil
- 1 teaspoon Himalayan salt
- 3 cups spinach
- ½ radicchio, thinly shredded
- 3 cups beets, peeled, chopped and roasted
- 1 cup red onion, diced
- 1 cup pomegranate seeds
- 2 tablespoons walnuts, toasted and crushed

Directions

1.   In a small bowl, whisk together the coconut aminos, vinegar, orange zest, orange juice, maple syrup, olive oil and salt.

2.   In a large salad bowl, toss together the spinach, radicchio, beets, red onion, and pomegranate seeds. Drizzle with dressing and toss to coat. Garnish with walnuts.

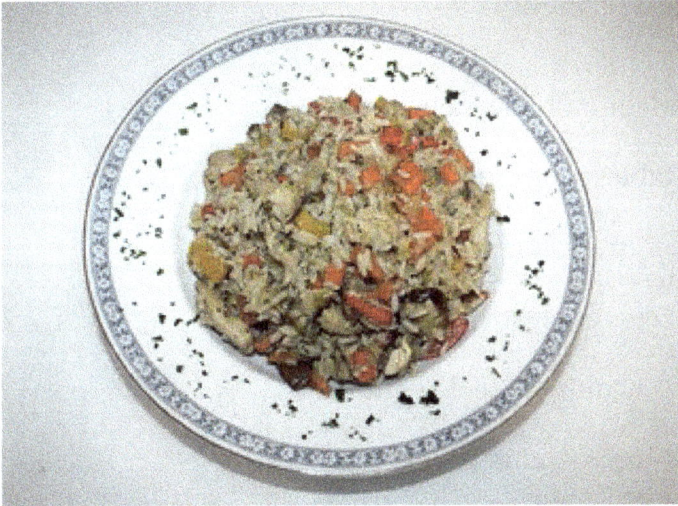

Sweet Summer Soup

Servings: 2

Total Time: 15 minutes

Ingredients

- 1 medium honeydew melon
- 2 tablespoons lemon juice
- ¼ cup fresh raspberries
- ¼ cup fresh strawberry
- ½ cucumber, peeled and diced
- ¼ cup coconut milk (from a can)

Directions

1. Place all ingredients, except the coconut milk in a blender and mix until smooth.

2. Pour into serving bowls and pour coconut milk into each as garnish.

Melon Pie

Servings: 2

Total Time: 15 minutes

Ingredients

- 4 circular slices of a small watermelon
- 1/3 cup unsweetened yogurt
- 3 kiwis, sliced
- ½ cup strawberries, sliced
- ¼ cup blueberries
- 10 grapes, halved
- ¼ teaspoon cinnamon
- 1 teaspoon raw honey
- 2 teaspoons mint leaves, chopped

Directions

1. Lay out watermelon slices and spread yogurt on each slice.

2. Top with kiwi, strawberries, blueberries and grapes. Sprinkle cinnamon on each slice.

3. Drizzle with honey and top each slice with mint leaves.

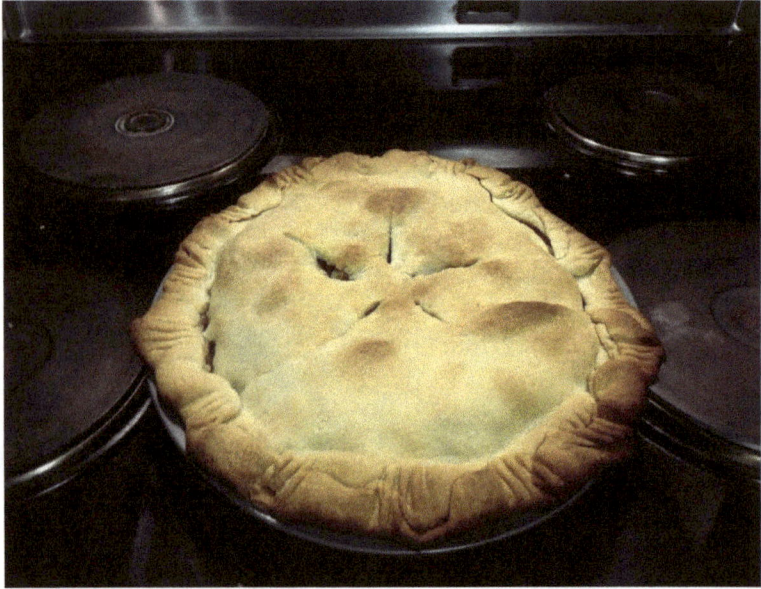

Super Smooth Parsnip Soup

Servings: 2

Total Time: 30 minutes

Ingredients

- ½ tablespoon olive oil

- 2 shallots, sliced

- 1 celery stalk, chopped

- 1 garlic clove, crushed

- 1 teaspoon fennel seeds

- 1 parsnip, chopped

- ¼ teaspoon cayenne pepper

- 2 cups vegetable stock

- ½ medium cauliflower head, cut into florets

- ½ teaspoon Himalayan salt

- ½ teaspoon black pepper, crushed

- 1 tablespoon green onions, sliced

Directions

1.   In a large saucepan over medium heat, add oil, shallots, celery, garlic and fennel seeds. Cook for 5 minutes or until softened. Add in parsnips and cayenne pepper. Cook 2 minutes.

2.   Add vegetable stock, cauliflower, salt and pepper. Bring to a low boil then reduce heat to low and simmer 15 minutes.

3.   Blend cooled soup in a blender or food processor until smooth. Reheat in a saucepan over medium heat. Ladle into bowl, garnish with green onions and serve.

Cucumber & Salmon Cups

Servings: 2

Total Time: 10 minutes

Ingredients

- 1 large cucumber, sliced into 1 ½ inch slices

- 10 - 12 smoked salmon pieces

- 10 - 12 dill fronds

- ½ tablespoon olive oil

- ½ teaspoon black pepper, crushed

Directions

1. For each cucumber slice, hollow out one end so that you can create a little cup.

2. Fold the smoked salmon piece enough so that you can fit it in the cucumber cup hole. Add a dill frond to each cup.

3. Drizzle with olive oil and sprinkle with black pepper.

Sweet Potato Toasts

Servings: 2

Total Time: 15 minutes

Ingredients

- 1 small sweet potato, sliced into 1 ½ inch slices

- ½ cup raspberries

- ½ lime, juiced

- 1 teaspoon lime zest

- 1 tablespoon chia seeds

- 3 tablespoons cashew butter

- 1 tablespoon pumpkin seeds, toasted

- 1 tablespoon raisins

Directions

1. Place sweet potato slices in griller and grill/toast on high until slightly browned.

2. In a small bowl, mash the raspberries along with the lime juice and zest. Stir in chia seeds and let sit for 10 minutes.

3.   Spread cashew butter on each slice of sweet potato. Then add the raspberry chia jam spread you created on each slice.

4.   Top with pumpkin seeds and raisins.

Eggplant Cashew Bites

Servings: 2

Total Time: 15 minutes

Ingredients

- 1 eggplant, very thinly sliced
- 1 tablespoon olive oil
- 1 teaspoon Himalayan salt
- 1 tablespoon pine nuts
- 1 tablespoon raisins

Cashew Basil Filling

- 1 cup cashews, soaked overnight and drained
- 1 lemon, juiced
- 3 tablespoons water
- 1 tablespoon nutritional yeast
- ½ teaspoon Himalayan salt
- ¼ teaspoon black pepper, crushed
- ¼ teaspoon ground nutmeg
- 1 handful fresh basil, roughly chopped

Directions

1.　　Place broiler on high and line a baking tray with parchment paper.

2.　　Brush each slice of eggplant with olive oil and season with salt. Place on the baking tray. Broil 4 minutes and then flip to broil 4 minutes on the other side.

3.　　Make Cashew Basil Filling by placing all ingredients in a food processor and blending until smooth.

4.　　Remove Cashew Basil Filling from food processor and mix in the pine nuts and raisins.

5.　　Place Cashew Basil Filling in each of the eggplant slices and roll up, securing with a toothpick. Serve immediately.

Curry Chips

Servings: 2

Total Time: 35 minutes

Ingredients

- 1 bunch curly kale, stems removed and torn into pieces

Curry Spice Mix

- 1 tablespoon melted coconut oil

- 1 tablespoon lemon juice

- 2 garlic cloves, minced

- 1 teaspoon turmeric

- 1 teaspoon red chili flakes

- 1 teaspoon Himalayan salt

- ½ teaspoon black pepper, crushed

- ¼ teaspoon ground ginger

- ¼ teaspoon coriander

- ¼ teaspoon cardamom

- ⅛ teaspoon cumin

Directions

1.   In a small bowl, combine the coconut oil, lemon juice, garlic, turmeric, chili flakes, salt, pepper, ginger, coriander, cardamom and cumin.

2.   Line two baking trays with parchment paper and preheat oven to 275°F/135°C.

3.   Pour Curry Spice Mix over all the kale and toss well to coat, ensuring spices get into every part of the kale leaves. Place kale on baking tray and place in the oven.

4.   Bake the kale chips for 30 minutes, rotating pans once.

Mexican Dip

Servings: 2

Total Time: 30 minutes

Ingredients

- 1 cup lentils, cooked
- 1 garlic clove, minced
- ½ teaspoon cumin
- ½ teaspoon Himalayan salt
- 2 tablespoons green onions, sliced

Salsa

- 1 tomato, diced
- ½ green bell pepper
- ½ red onion, diced
- ½ lime, squeezed
- 1 tablespoon cilantro, chopped

Yogurt

- 1 cup unsweetened goat yogurt
- ½ teaspoon cumin

- ½ teaspoon cayenne pepper

Guacamole

- 1 avocado

- 1 garlic clove, grated

- 1 jalapeno, seeded and diced

- ½ red onion, diced

- ½ teaspoon Himalayan salt

Directions

1. Make base layer by combining lentils, 1 garlic clove, ½ teaspoon cumin and ½ teaspoon salt in a small bowl. Spread on the bottom of a small glass baking dish. Make salsa layer by combining the all the salsa ingredients together in a bowl. Place this mixture on top of the lentils.

2. Using another bowl, whip together the yogurt ingredients and place on top of the salsa.

3. In a small bowl, mash together the guacamole ingredients to make the guacamole. Spread on top of the yogurt layer.

4. Garnish with green onions and serve with cut up vegetables.

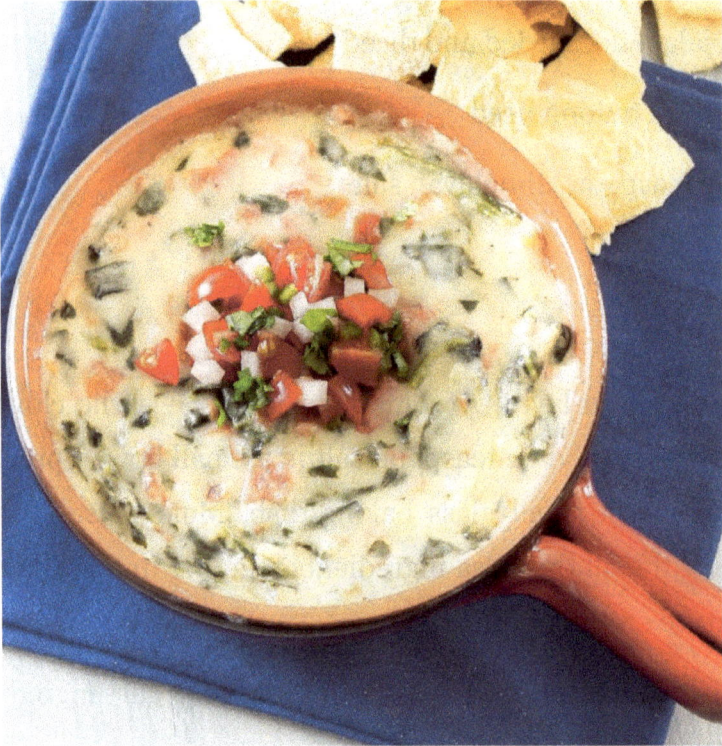

www.ingramcontent.com/pod-product-compliance
Lightning Source LLC
Chambersburg PA
CBHW062342300326
41947CB00012B/1181